Introduction

In March of 2007 I was diagnosed with a mental illness.

I wrote this book to help others understand what it's like to live with and understand my mental illness...it is called Schizoaffective Disorder.

Table of Contents

Schizoaffective Disorder

What Is It   4

Schizophrenia

    Symptoms   5

    Hallucinations   6

    Delusions   7

    Thought Disorder   8

Bipolar Disorder

    Mania   9

    Depression   10

    Mood Changes   11

Hygiene   12

Medication   13

Therapy   14

Stress   15

Support   16

Sleep   17

Exercise   17

Steps to help Recovery   18

My Story   19

Thank You   23

What is Schizoaffective Disorder?

Schizoaffective Disorder is a mental illness that is found in people who have both Schizophrenia and a mood disorder like Bipolar Disorder or Depression.

The American Psychiatrist John Kasanin has been said to introduce the term Schizoaffective Disorder on 1933. Originally it was called Schizoaffective Psychosis.

Schizoaffective Disorder is hard to diagnose and get treatment for because it is a combination of to mental illnesses. Often people get misdiagnosed as one of the disorders or the other and not get proper treatment. The disorder usually appears in people when they are in their late teens or in early adulthood.

Schizophrenia

Schizophrenia is defined as a disorder that causes a person to lose touch with reality.

Symptoms

- Hallucinations and Delusions- Seeing things that aren't there
- Thought Disorder- Words that don't come out right
- Disorganized Behavior- inappropriate emotions in situations
- Loss of Intrest in every day activities
- Lack of emotion
- Reduced ability to plan or carry out activities
- Neglect of personal hygiene
- Social withdrawal
- No motivation
- Problems with making sense of information
- Difficulty paying attention
- Memory problems.

Hallucinations

Hallucinations can come in many ways; through taste, touch, sight, and/or hearing. The most common form of hallucinations is hearing voices that aren't really there.

The voices a person may hear with Schizophrenia can be so real to the person that whatever the voices tell them to do, like harm themselves, they will do it. The voices can also comment on the person's daily activities and give the him or her a sense of being defeated by taunting the inflicted.

There may be more than one voice talking at the same time or the voices will talk to each other creating too much noise inside your head. They love to comment on how stupid or worthless a person is.

Sometimes the voices can be happy and a joy to have around, like friends, but only to stab you in the back later by mean comments

Delusions

Delusions are false beliefs held by the schizophrenic person. No matter how hard you try to convince them that the thoughts or beliefs aren't real, that it is all in their head, they do not give up the fact that they believe they are real. For example there are paranoid delusions and delusions of persecution. An example of the types I just said would be that people are "out to get you" or the thoughts that people are doing things behind your back like talking about you when in reality the people may just be knitting or reading a book.

Other types of Delusions are that of Reference. Delusions of Reference are when things in the environment seem to be directly related to you, even though they are not. An example of this would be that it may seem as if people are talking about you or to you personally about special messages hidden through the wave lengths of the TV set.

There are other types of delusions but those are the most common. To the person with Schizophrenia these thoughts are very real and true. Schizophrenic people have a very hard time distinguishing between reality and imagination.

Thought Disorder

A common disorder in the brain of a person with schizophrenia is called Thought Disorder. This is best explained when the person tries to talk and they get confused on what they are trying to say. The thoughts are scrambled and the person can't get the thoughts into a spoken language.

Sometimes the thoughts come out but they come out in the wrong order; instead of saying "look at the cat eating a fish" it would come out as "look a cat at the fish is eating a." This is the most frustrating part of the disorder to deal with. Nobody understands what you are thinking or what you are trying to say. You end up repeating yourself until the thought comes out correctly.

Another part of the Thought Disorder is when you are talking and in mid-sentence your mind goes blank like a clean slate and the story or thought you were telling is completely gone and you don't even know what you were talking about it's like the whole story or thought disappeared from your mind. When this happens the person listening to you gets lost in what you were saying, wondering what the next word is, trying to help you but the conversation stops and you go onto something totally different.

Bipolar Disorder

Bipolar Disorder is defined as a mental illness where a person experiences mood changes from euphoria to depression.

Mania symptoms

- Euphoria and Extreme Optimism
- Inflated Self-Esteem
- Poor Judgment and Risky Behavior
- Rapid Speech and Racing Thoughts
- Aggressive Behavior
- Irritation

- Increased Physical Activity
- Spending Sprees or Unwise Financial Choices
- Increased Drive to Perform or Achieve Goals
- Increased Sex Drive
- Decreased Need for Sleep
- Inability to Concentrate
- Careless or Dangerous Use of Drugs or Alcohol
- Frequent Absences and/or Poor Performance at Work or School
- Delusions or a break from reality (psychosis)

Depression

Depression is also found in Bipolar Disorder. Here are the Symptoms of Depression

- Sadness and Hopelessness
- Suicidal Thoughts or Behavior
- Anxiety
- Guilt
- Sleep Problems
- Low Appetite or Increased Appetite
- Fatigue
- Loss of Interest in Daily Activities
- Problems Concentrating

- Irritability
- Chronic Pain without a Known Cause
- Frequent Absences from Work or School
- Poor Performance at Work or School

Mood changes

Earlier I said that a person with Schizoaffective Disorder means that they have both Schizophrenia and Bipolar Disorder or Depression. The person with Schizoaffective Disorder also experiences mood changes. These changes include depression which means that you are very sad and nothing can cheer you up. You can also experience Mania which is the feeling being overly happy, being really excited, having racing thoughts and having a whole bunch of crazy ideas for no apparent reason. You can also experience Hypomania which is a lesser degree of Mania, or a mixture of both moods at the same time.

Swings in mood changes vary from person to person. Some people may experience one to two episodes of Mania, Depression or both at the same time within 12 months.

Other mood changes could be switching four or more times within 12 months this is called Rapid Cycling. Ultra Rapid Cycling is when a person changes moods every couple of days.

Another fast mood changing cycle is called Ultra-Ultra Rapid Cycling. This cycle is when you have numerous mood changes in one day.

The final type of fast cycle is called Ultradian Rapid Cycling. The moods switch from a few minutes to a few hours before switching to a different mood again.

Hygiene

The person with Schizoaffective Disorder lacks the ability to take care of themselves. The most troubled areas are showering, bathing, brushing own hair and keeping their teeth brushed.

The caregiver(s) need to remind or keep a schedule for the person to help track what days to take showers. A note on a mirror is a good tool for reminding the person to brush their hair and teeth every day

Medication

Schizoaffective people need a variety of medication to be able to live in the general population. The medication that is most effective includes anti-psychotics, mood stabilizers and anti-depressants. Sometimes anti-anxiety medication and anti-convulsants are also prescribed by a psychiatrist.

Some medication brand names include Geodon, Invega, and Risperdal these are anti-psychotics. Lithium and Prozac are effective mood stabilizers and Clonazepam and Lorazepam, may be used for anti-anxiety medication. Trileptal is an anti-convulsant. Anti-convulsants are sometimes used because they can help control the chemical imbalances in a person's brain.

It is a slow process to get the right combination of medicine. The patient needs to work closely with their psychiatrist and follow the directions to a "T". It is a trial and error period for perfecting the combination as everyone is different.

Having the correct combination is such a relief. Once the patient is reacting to a specific combination, they will feel like they are back to where they can function and act relatively normal.

Again, I need to stress that it takes a few weeks for the medicine to get into your system and begin working effectively - so you have to be patient.

The patient also needs to expect a few adjustments along the way, but once the right combination of medication is working, be sure to continue using it for the rest of your life.

Therapy

Therapy is something that is very important and is a must have for people with Schizoaffective Disorder. The psychiatrist will make a recommendation of a psychologist who is experienced in your illness.

Therapy can help the patient express personal feelings about the disorder. Therapy also helps the patient cope in realizing that they have a life long illness and guides the person to get back on track just like before they developed the disorder. Therapy can also help reduce stress by giving a person with Schizoaffective

Disorder techniques to cope with the stress of everyday life.

The therapist will help the person by teaching them to do breathing exercises, listening to your inner thoughts, slow and calm your mind, and to sit in a bubble type visualization meditation exercise that will help with stress and racing thoughts.

Stress

I cannot tell you how important it is for a schizoaffective person to not have stress in their lives. Stress is a major trigger for symptoms and the symptoms can come back even though they are under control with the right combination of medication. Stress can also make the symptoms worse. Depending on the severity of the disorder, it might mean that a person can handle more stress then say another person with the schizoaffective disorder.

Support

Support is another huge factor when getting back to being able to function. Family is the best support for a person who has any mental illness in general.

Family members are the loving caregivers. They play an important role in reminding the person to take their medication on-time every day and let the doctor know when they need an adjustment. They also need to keep tabs on the hygiene.

They can also help by reassuring the person that things are going to be alright and that they love them unconditionally. This really is important when they are in a depressed mood. The family will need to reassure them if they are having delusions and/or hallucinations by saying what they are thinking and seeing isn't real and that no one can harm them and that they are safe.

Animals can also play a part in supporting the schizoaffective patient by always being there for the person. The person can feel comfortable around the animal and not worry about being judged. Animals always listen and don't mind being talked to, held and petted. I have also found that animals have a calming effect on my disorder.

Sleep

To help combat the effects of the Schizoaffective Disorder, a person needs to get a lot of sleep. Sleep is very important, if you don't get enough sleep, your mood could switch between depression, mania or even hypomania.

Sleep also gives the physical body time to regenerate, let the medicine work and it lets your mind get much needed rest. For me, I need between 12 and 14 hours of sleep a night and if I get anything less than 12 hours of sleep my mood switches during the day between depression, mania and hypomania.

EXERCISE

Exercise helps a lot, especially when it comes to needing to focus on stuff like school work and it helps to clear your mind and shut off the voices.

When I am really stressed out, I find that taking a walk helps me un-stress, relaxes me and just makes my mind so much clearer than before.

STEPS TO HELP RECOVERY

I read these steps daily – they help me cope with the illness.

- Accept that you have a prolonged illness
- Identify your strengths and limitations
- Make clear, realistic goals
- After a relapse, go slowly and gradually back to your responsibilities
- Plan a regular, consistent and predictable daily routine
- Make your home a quiet, calm and relaxed haven
- Identify and reduce stress
- Make one change at a time in your life
- Work towards an active and trusting relationship
- Take medications regularly and as prescribed
- Make your own warning list
- Get involved in a group that makes you feel comfortable

- Avoid street drugs, alcohol and eat a well-balanced diet
- Get enough rest and regular exercise
- If you lose sight of reality, ask for help to bring you back
- Accept setbacks and don't get discouraged

My Story

Before I was diagnosed as having Schizoaffective Disorder, I would skip school a lot because I couldn't handle the stress of getting all the homework done and having it done by a specific date. I would "pretend" to be "sick" although some days I actually was sick. Most of the time, I just couldn't deal with the homework. This went on for about 2 years.

In 9th grade, I finally broke down and basically lost it. I freaked out so bad because someone made up a song about me and I became very angry and told the other person I was going to kill him. After that the school counselor told my parents that I needed psychiatric help. So half-way through 9th grade, I met my psychiatrist.

Before I could get help through medication, I had to see a psychologist for testing to see what kind of disorder I had. Before the testing the psychologist wrote down a family history of illnesses from talking with my mom. After the history was written down I began testing. The tests that were done included looking at ink blots and describing what I saw. I also had to take a very long descriptive personality test that was over 400 questions long. It took me, I think, 4 hours to complete and a normal person could complete it in 1 - 2 hours. It took me that long because I was so out of reality and would space out and have to get back in reality to finish the test.

I then had another appointment with my psychiatrist. At this appointment, my test results were in and the psychologist wrote a report of what he found out about me and what disorder I had. In March of 2007, I was officially diagnosed as having Schizoaffective Disorder Bipolar Type. This diagnosis helped explain everything that was going on in my life.

My Psychiatrist began trying out combinations of medication to take away the delusions and hallucinations. This required my mom to take me to office visits once a week until the medication worked. I couldn't control my feelings or my life – I was out of control, needing a huge amount of time and support from my family.

The delusions I had were very bizarre but somewhat common with Schizophrenia. I say the delusions were common because I was paranoid and had delusions about aliens. I had thoughts of aliens sucking out my brain, giant whales eating people, and people looking at me or talking about me when I walked into a room and even people secretly planning against me.

I also had thoughts that if I was to drink liquid through a straw, the aliens were hiding in the straw and they would launch into my brain and get me. Another thought was that fridgerator magnets were secretly vampires and could fly and bite me.

The hallucinations I had were hearing voices that told me to not take my medicine. I could even hear multiple voices talking really loud at the same time I was seeing aliens and people crawling on the ceiling, along with severed heads on counters. I saw people and huge animals peering in at me through the windows. At one point I heard very tiny people talking to me and laughing at me. But all that slowly started to disappear.

After the medication controlled the hallucinations and delusions, my first mood switching episodes started. The switching was very slow, like maybe once or twice a month then it slowly got worse.

Currently my mood switches between once every few days (Ultra Rapid Cycling) to multiple times a day (Ultradian Rapid Cycling). I can go from being Manic to Depressed in an instant at any time. I have recently came to the conclusion and realization that I am always in a Hypomanic state. From the minute I wake up to the time I go to bed I am non-stop chatter. The only time I am not talking for any length of time is when I get really tired then I become mute.

Having Schizoaffective Disorder has made me aware of my thoughts and feelings. I can now tell when my mood switches to some degree but for the most part, I am under control.

I have made major improvements over the last 5 years. I went from no eye contact when speaking to someone, to actually looking at the person in the eyes when in a conversation. I used to speak in a monotone voice, no expression and a lifeless dull look to being happy and totally full of expression.

It has been a long road for me and my family; I have made future goals and have found a new side to life.

In reading my book I hope you or someone you may know may be enlightened by what I have told you and will know that there are others like you. Do not be afraid or feel like an outcast, just know that you aren't alone.

My Thanks

I want to take this opportunity to thank my family and friends. You have all helped me in my life and this illness. A special thank you to:

Dr. Patric Darby, psychiatrist

Without this support, I wouldn't be who I am today

Thank you.

www.ingramcontent.com/pod-product-compliance
Lightning Source LLC
Chambersburg PA
CBHW071605170526
45166CB00004B/1800